T0365628

THE ADDICTION CONSPIRACY

Unlocking Brain Chemistry and Addiction so
You Don't Have to Struggle

Lee Tannenbaum, M.D.

AuthorHouse™
1663 Liberty Drive
Bloomington, IN 47403
www.authorhouse.com
Phone: 833-262-8899

Because of the dynamic nature of the Internet, any web addresses or links contained in this book may have changed since publication and may no longer be valid. The views expressed in this work are solely those of the author and do not necessarily reflect the views of the publisher, and the publisher hereby disclaims any responsibility for them.

Any people depicted in stock imagery provided by Getty Images are models, and such images are being used for illustrative purposes only. Certain stock imagery © Getty Images.

This book is printed on acid-free paper.

ISBN: 978-1-4343-6648-1 (sc)

Library of Congress Control Number: 2008900771

Print information available on the last page.

Published by AuthorHouse 06/24/2022

authorHOUSE®

This book is dedicated to my patients at the Bel Air Center for Addictions who demonstrate the daily courage to control their disease and lead a normal, happy life in the face of adversity. Your stories are inspiring. May they help others to reclaim their lives from the disease of addiction.

Acknowledgments

I gratefully acknowledge and thank all the speakers and other experts in the field of addiction who shared their knowledge with me at various seminars, conferences, symposiums and other meetings. These individuals taught me about the disease of addiction and it was their enthusiasm, passion, and willingness to share their knowledge that inspired me to begin my own practice. Much of the content of this book comes from what others taught me. I utilized information they provided me to do the best I could to explain some of the underlying concepts of addiction so non-medical people would be able to understand them. This book is the combination of personal notes and experiences and I apologize if I inadvertently included any direct information from someone else without proper acknowledgement.

Addiction is a very complicated disease and the information in this book is presented in the form of simplified models for illustrative purposes. The concepts presented are the important thing. The details, particularly in this rapidly evolving field where extensive research is always in progress, may be less than accurate and frankly, may have already been proven inaccurate by the time this comes to print.

Nonetheless, I believe this book will allow most readers to gain a significant understanding of the underlying concepts of the neurochemistry of addiction and the implications for treatment options. If any reader desires more detailed or comprehensive information, I would refer them to a number of excellent and extensive textbooks and more current articles on the topic.

I also wish to thank my family, friends and co-workers for all their support in this effort, particularly my wife Debbie and my daughters, Lisa and Amy. Special thanks to my friend Katlyn who never had to struggle.

Foreword: What You Think You Know

Everyone thinks they know about addiction. Whether or not you've ever popped a pill or used a needle, everyone thinks they know about drugs, the types of people addicted to them and how those people should overcome their addiction. What people think they know about addiction correlates directly to how society tells them to think about addiction. Is addiction a disease or a behavior? And, does it matter how addiction is being treated?

The politically correct answer is, of course, that addiction is a disease. Do most people really believe that? Despite the fact that many people, if asked, will respond that addiction is a disease, there are not many people who really adhere to this idea.

This book challenges how we, as a society, think about addiction and how those suffering from the disease of addiction think about themselves. It is not productive for us to continue to kick those who are down and to tell them they've been bad. Understanding brain chemistry proves once and for all it's not their fault and they don't have to struggle to lead normal, happy, productive lives. There is hope. There is help.

Chapter 1: Journey to Addiction Medicine

I had always been a social, albeit heavy, drinker – a couple of beers every night after work and then pour it on over the weekend. At some point about three years ago I decided that I was drinking too much and was going to slow down. I couldn't. It scared me, so I decided to quit completely for a period of time, but I couldn't do that either. Suddenly, I found myself drinking vodka first thing in the morning and throughout the day. I would pour vodka into water bottles and hide them all over the house and garage. I'd drink from the bottles in the liquor cabinet but I always made sure to fill them back up so my wife didn't notice that they were getting lower. My addiction was so bad that I literally could not function without alcohol in my system.

I believe that my body got to a point where it needed to be around .12 or so in order for me to function to what I considered to be normal. Toward the very end, my routine was to get up at around 4 a.m., walk downstairs and take a shot or two so I could stop shaking, and go back to sleep. I'd wake up around 7 a.m., take a couple more shots and off to work. Work for a couple of hours, go to lunch and take a couple of shots. Once the day finally ended, then I was "free" to drink because that was considered normal. I'd have a few beers and of course sneak shots in here and there. At this point I was already drunk but nobody really noticed.

◈

After about a year of using heroin, I was spending every dime I made on it. I went from being a successful horse trainer and loving mother to a miserable, very sick woman with absolutely nothing.

◈

My addiction took about two years of my life away from me. It started out somewhat manageable but quickly became very hard to maintain mentally, physically and financially. My addiction was big enough to rule every second of every day of my life for that time period. It became a 24-hour a day job of worrying about how and where my next fix was going to come from – that is literally all I cared about.

I got involved in addiction medicine by accident. I personally have never been touched by the disease of addiction. I have never had an addicted child. I have never been dependent on any substance. I have never been an alcoholic. I did not set out from the very beginning determined to fix the lives of those ravaged by addiction.

When one of the most well-known addiction treatment centers in the world, which happened to bc located close to my home, needed a part-time physician, I agreed to perform physical exams on patients at the time of their admission and provide medical services if they became ill during their inpatient stay. Other staff members handled the addiction treatment program and while I knew they managed a strict 28-day inpatient program based on abstinence and the twelve steps, I did not know much about the specifics of addiction treatment.

After 10 years at this internationally-recognized facility, the director provided my name as a reference to another inpatient addiction center in the area. They needed someone to fill in while their medical director was on leave for health reasons. I began working at this facility part-time in 2001. It was here, though, that I met a new challenge: In addition to patients' routine medical issues, I was expected to know more about how to treat their addictions.

I decided to read the Big Book, the "bible" of Alcoholics Anonymous and the basis for all twelve-step addiction treatment programs. This was the treatment used at both facilities where I had gained experience and apparently was the standard of care everywhere. As a family physician, I had also referred many patients for this type of program. I wondered exactly what the Big Book had to say so I decided, quite simply, to find out.

To sum up my reaction, I was shocked. I had been searching for a sensible, medical approach to treating addiction, but the book assured me this wasn't possible. Apparently, the standard of addiction treatment was to ask patients to turn their lives over to a higher power and be healed! I found out that addicts and alcoholics really were hopeless and now I understood why I had never learned anything about addiction treatment; there was nothing to learn. Neither was there any medical support to offer these patients.

According to the Big Book, those poor miserable souls who unfortunately had become addicted to drugs or alcohol needed to learn to make better choices. This condition had very little to do with medicine or real diseases. It seemed counseling from psychologists could offer some hope or maybe a psychiatric evaluation could diagnose and treat depression, but if these people continued to ***choose*** to use drugs or alcohol, what could we really do for them?

Despite the lack of information, I took my position as medical director of an addiction facility, albeit temporary, very seriously. I also needed 50 hours of continuing medical education per year to keep my board certification and license. So, the next time I saw an addiction conference offered, I decided to go.

Many patients describe addiction medicine as life changing. Learning about addiction medicine was life changing for me as a physician. For the first time, I interacted with other physicians who discussed the science of addiction as a disease. Most interestingly, the information presented about addiction was similar to information I had learned about other diseases – theories of causes, statistics about prevalence and incidence, physiology, biochemistry, and even thoughts about medical treatments. Certainly, there was ample discussion about the role of twelve-step, abstinence-based programs and how they supplemented addiction medicine. However, these were discussed as one of *several* tools physicians could use to treat *patients* with the *disease* of addiction. Yes, they were patients rather than simply addicts, and the goal was to help them manage their disease so they could lead happy, productive lives just like every other patient. Where had all this information been all of my professional life?

Chapter 2: Addicts or Patients?

Like most people, I tried a methadone program. This was not effective at all and even made things worse for me. It was at the methadone clinic where I met a fellow addict who introduced me to heroin and needles. Most people I encountered at the clinic were still using. It was horrible. They were abusing both street opiates and methadone… it was easy to score drugs there and to talk other people into getting high again. Despite all of this, even before I relapsed with heroin, the methadone was not controlling my cravings at all. It just made me feel doped up and tired. I literally would get my dose in the morning and come home and sleep most of the day away. This went on for about eight months and it was almost as bad as using. More bad came out of the methadone program than good.

◈

I went to a 10-day rehab where they gave medication to help me sleep for the first three days. The next seven days there were classes all day long. You felt like shit, you didn't sleep, you had trouble eating. It was rough. It was like what you think that going through detox would be like. It took a lot of willpower to do that and stay there.

◈

It's not a personal weakness and I'm not a bad person because I do it. I'm not weak and lacking self control.

Once I learned about addiction medicine, I truly had a new focus in life. I was the first guy on my block with new and fascinating information about this disease that was surrounding us. What I found out next was an even greater shock to me; no one in my medical circles wanted to hear about this fascinating new information or wanted to know anything about addiction.

I experienced firsthand the stigma my patients deal with on a daily basis. The stigma that follows many people who suffer from addiction is well embedded in society, including many of my colleagues in the medical field. They see addicts as dirty, weak-minded individuals that use alcohol or drugs only to get high. The stigma classifies addicts as criminals, degenerates, and spouse abusers and often as destitute and homeless. Addicts aren't considered sick, just bad.

Most people, despite what they might have heard or read, think addiction to drugs or alcohol is a behavior under the addict's control. It is easy to see why we believe this without looking at the scientific evidence. After all, if someone were to hold a gun to an addict's head and tell him that if he used he would be shot, the drug addict would be able to turn down the drug in order to save his own life. Compare this to something we know is a disease – say, diabetes. If someone were to hold a gun to a diabetic's head and command him to lower his blood sugar on the spot or be killed, the diabetic would be unable to, no matter how much he wished or tried.

This is how people tend to view the difference between behavior and disease; a disease is completely and totally out of the patient's control while a behavior, if the motivation is strong enough, can be started or stopped on command. Addiction certainly looks like a behavior, and for decades it has been widely believed that addicts can stop using if the motivation to do so is strong enough. This seems logical, but like most things that seem obvious to the naked eye, there is another much more complicated explanation beneath the surface.

This explanation is beginning to come to light as addiction is just starting to be better understood by science. We now know more about addiction than we ever have in the past, but that knowledge hasn't yet been widely accepted and myths have sprung up in its place. It's time we examine some of those myths and talk about the new, real scientific knowledge that has risen up to debunk them. Let's look at our perception of addiction and its victims, and tell the truth.

The most common perception of an addict is of someone smoking crack or shooting heroin in a back alley. This is a particularly poisonous myth concerning addiction and it has crept into every aspect of how we deal with the disease. Look at the words that we use when we discuss addiction. Addicts are "dirty" when they are using and "clean" when they are not. These terms have been influenced by the ideas that addicts can control their own behavior and that addicts live in poverty and squalor with their drugs. Terms like "dirty" and "clean" have come to be labels that carry with them significant moral judgments that support the behavioral theory of addiction. We don't tell diabetics that they are "dirty" when their blood sugar is high. Why should the person who suffers from the disease of addiction be morally judged any differently when his disease is out of control?

This stereotype is reinforced in every fiber of our society. Unfortunately, it seems that many people who are knowledgeable about addiction treatment secretly believe this, even if they tacitly tow the party line that "addiction is a disease." They all know, really deep down, that most addicts probably deserve their lot in life and they could get better if they really wanted. Many people continue to believe that addiction is a self-inflicted problem, or a voluntary behavior, and that appropriate education, motivation, and willpower of the addicted person will result in effective treatment. This is the biggest myth of all, and the worst part about it is that those who spread it simply don't know any better. They themselves fall victim to the same ignorance and fear of change that they assign to drug addicts.

Society dictates that these bad, dirty addicts need to go to jail or to AA to pledge their lives to abstinence and get clean. If they were unsuccessful in these programs, they might have to go to methadone maintenance, that black hole where drug addicts go when they are no longer suitable to live in society like the rest of us. Many of my colleagues thought that they were not seeing patients with addiction problems in their practices. They believed that bums and vagrants, who drug addicts invariably were, didn't come into a respectable doctor's office unless they were trying to con the physicians out of prescription drugs that they could misuse or sell. While many people gave lip service to the politically correct idea that addiction is a disease, I couldn't find anyone who truly believed this.

As I learned at addiction treatment conferences and through additional research and education, there is information and evidence we can use to combat the myths and treat addiction for what it truly is – a disease. As I first started learning about addiction medicine, a new medication, buprenorphine, was approved as an opioid addiction treatment prescribed out of a physician's office, rather than in the typical established drug treatment centers. I was familiar with buprenorphine. At the centers where I worked, it was the primary drug used to detoxify patients when they came in addicted to narcotic drugs. Buprenorphine was prescribed for three to five days with a goal of relieving patients' most severe withdrawal symptoms. It was then always discontinued as patients were moved to the main abstinence-based treatment portion of the programs.

Allowing buprenorphine to be prescribed from a physician's office was an attempt to promote the idea of maintenance therapy rather than short term "detox" therapies and to expand the idea of maintenance therapy beyond methadone clinics. It certainly was a safe enough drug to prescribe out of my office, so I decided to give it a try. I took the required training course and received my certification to prescribe the medication. With some trepidation about really deciding to see "those" types of patients in my nice office, I allowed my name to be placed on the buprenorphine provider Web site and soon thereafter scheduled my first addiction patient.

Chapter 3: Change Your Life Overnight - One Patient's Story

Each story is different, yet so similar. Each patient I meet carries the burden and desperation of an addiction that has ruined their lives or stands at the cusp of losing it all. Patients suffering from the disease of addiction are everywhere, including in the most seemingly normal households.

John's story might be your story. John's story might be your brother's story or your father's or your friend's. When I met John in April 2003, his story sounded like one I had heard many times before. He sounded typical, in one way or another, to all the addicts I had ever admitted to the rehab facility where I worked. It was seldom anyone's first time being admitted for treatment. Everyone always sincerely wanted to quit using, even though they just seemed unable to make the commitment to do so. I was not very hopeful that this time would be any different for John and I fully expected to probably never see him again.

At age 40, John identified himself as a recovering alcoholic. He had been sober from alcohol since 1989, but explained that he had a severe and ongoing addiction to heroin. He had been using about $100 worth of heroin a day for the past two years. John had tried rehab several times since 1989, but never stayed very long, as he was unable to get past the severe withdrawal symptoms that plagued him when he stopped using. John noted that in the past two years his longest period of time without using had been five days. John was an active member of AA but he admitted he was never really honest when he was there. He had last used earlier the same morning he saw me and he did not want to go back to another rehab program. After a careful evaluation, I prescribed buprenorphine for John and advised him to see me again the next day.

To my surprise, John not only showed up for his visit the next day, but he was actually better! He was feeling okay and had only minimal withdrawal symptoms. He also had a good outlook on continuing his treatment with me. John stated that he was very happy with the treatment program so far and he felt as if he had been given a new lease on life. Let me emphasize again that this was *one day* into the treatment program for a relatively hard-core addict, battling opiate addiction almost his entire adult life. I was pretty amazed and encouraged. We continued his treatment.

I next saw John two days later. This time, John noted he was not feeling sick; in fact, he felt good overall and had no cravings or desire to use narcotics. He also realized that he did not feel depressed for the first time in months and he was very happy that he was saving a great deal of money by not having to support his drug habit. According to John, his mind was clear for the first time in years and he was finding that he did not have to plan out his days in advance based on when he was going to need his next fix. In a nutshell, John was pretty much cured. In three days, he transformed from a dead-end drug addict to a reasonably functioning person in society – all from a tiny pill.

I cannot stress enough the profound impact of John's miraculous recovery. I had been treating drug addicts for almost 10 years and I never saw a recovery like this. In fact, I never saw a recovery like this in any of my patients regardless of their disease. This treatment was truly a miracle. I found the answer to the scourge of drug addiction. I needed to tell everyone.

In an effort to reach other people like John in my community, I wrote an article for the local newspaper suggesting that perhaps there were other methods available and other ideas regarding addiction treatment. Perhaps it wasn't responsible medical treatment to exclusively recommend that everyone attend a twelve-step treatment program. The day after the article appeared in the paper, I received a phone call from the medical director of the world-renowned, abstinence-based addiction facility where I worked for 10 years. She fired me on the spot. Apparently, not only did no one want to hear about medical theories about addiction and their successes with treatment, but suggesting the idea that medical professionals might want to discuss the possibility of alternatives to twelve step programs was sacrilegious and unacceptable.

John remains drug-free after four years of buprenorphine maintenance and is the model of successful treatment. He continues to do well and he now owns two businesses. He is working hard, raising his family, taking care of his employees, paying his taxes and contributing to society. Several times, John considered trying to discontinue his maintenance therapy, but with each attempt, he felt the recurrence of cravings to use narcotics again and wisely chose to continue with his medication rather than jeopardize his recovery. Furthermore, John's miraculous story of recovery has been repeated literally hundreds of times in hundreds of other patients. John is not unique. Medical treatment is the key to overcoming the disease of addiction.

Chapter 4: The Missing Step in 12-Step Programs

Up to this point, I've discussed the concept of twelve-step programs only briefly. These strategies, which include Alcoholics Anonymous among others, have been the major foundation for addiction treatment for more than seventy years (Appendix A). They are not bad treatments. Twelve-step communities can form very supportive environments to help people suffering from addiction, who often feel that they are alone and shunned by society. Many addicts find relief in twelve-step programs and participants in these programs lead full and productive lives.

However, twelve-step programs are often misrepresented as the be-all and end-all in addiction treatment to the exclusion of all other options. Twelve-step programs have been painted as the only possible treatment of addiction and they have become almost cult-like institutions by fervent preaching of the myth that going through one of these programs is the only way to attain "true healing." Twelve-step programs continue to treat addiction as a behavior with moral shortcomings rather than a disease, so they produce a consistent failure rate despite their successes. It was never meant to be this way.

The Alcoholics Anonymous Big Book, outlining the twelve steps to recovery for alcoholics, was first published in 1939, almost 70 years ago. The twelve steps were developed simply because, at the time, medical science could not find any other effective treatment for alcoholism. The *symptoms* of addiction and the behaviors of taking drugs were well known back then as they are today, but the neurochemical *causes* of the disease were not. The twelve-step process was a treatment for the behavior and not the disease, but it was the only treatment of any kind that existed.

The introductory letter to the Big Book was penned by William D. Silkworth, a well-known doctor and chief physician at a prominent hospital specializing in alcohol and drug addiction. Dr. Silkworth recalled when in 1934, one year after the repeal of Prohibition, an alcoholic patient of his who had previously failed two courses of treatment "commenced to present his conceptions to other alcoholics, impressing upon them that they must do likewise with still others." He then noted that this became the basis of a rapidly growing fellowship of these men and their families. Dr. Silkworth's patient, and hundreds of others, appeared to recover from their disease. This was the birth of Alcoholics Anonymous, the oldest and most famous twelve-step program in existence.

However, if we continue to read Dr. Silkworth's letter, we note that he never thought this was the only treatment of this disease. In fact, Dr. Silkworth quite remarkably predicted the future. He began with the idea that alcoholics are "allergic" to alcohol and that, unlike most "normal" people, once they develop an addiction to it, they could never safely use alcohol again. He did not hold to the belief that alcoholism was primarily a problem of mental control, as he recognized the phenomenon of craving as common to all alcoholics. He recognized that in alcoholics, these cravings overrode all other interests so people continued to drink, not to escape or to seek euphoria, but because their cravings were beyond their mental control.

Unfortunately, Dr. Silkworth did not have the medical science at that time to locate the seat of this craving or to treat it effectively. He was only able to hypothesize that these cravings might be the manifestation of some kind of allergy which had never been permanently eradicated by any treatment available at that time. He felt that more than human power was needed to produce an essential psychic change to overcome the cravings and he noted that many alcoholics did not respond to ordinary psychological approaches. The only relief he could suggest was complete abstinence and he offered the stories of a group of his patients who believed in a Power which pulled them back from the gates of death as a way to attain this abstinence. In 1939, it was also noted that "Physicians who are familiar with alcoholism agree that there is no such thing as making a normal drinker out of an alcoholic. Science may one day accomplish this, but it hasn't done it yet."[1] This statement was true in 1939, three years before the first effective use of penicillin. Science has come a long way since then.

Craving is the key. Let's look at the problem stated earlier. The addict with a gun to his head can choose not to use his favorite drug and perhaps people would conclude that the addict can control his behavior and thus control his addiction. However, consider the real disease to be the underlying craving to use and not the use of the addictive substance itself. Even with a gun to his head, the addicted individual will still *want* to use. Yes, he can choose not to for a while, with the threat of imminent death hanging over his head. However, as time goes on and the immediate threat subsides, the cravings will eventually control the behavior and he will use again.

Seventy years after Dr. Silkworth's letter, we have a much more sophisticated understanding of neurobiology and have located the source and mechanism of these cravings that control addictive behavior - information which could only be guessed at in 1939.

Not only have we discovered the cause of addiction, we developed medications that get to the root of the cravings and treat them effectively. Abstinence and twelve step programs are not bad; they are just no longer the only option available. In many situations, and in fact most situations, addictive cravings can be controlled with medication and addictive behaviors can be changed with or without a twelve-step program.

If all of this is true, why aren't these medicines everywhere in the media and in the medical community? Why do twelve-step programs still exist, let alone in such rampant numbers? Why haven't you heard of this new treatment before? Why did I have to write a book about it at all – shouldn't something this wonderful speak for itself?

We could only hope. But the twelve-step program community has taken on a life of its own and it continues to resist the introduction of medications into its treatment programs. This is perhaps understandable given that these new discoveries disprove all of their treatment theories. However, the downside to this thinking is that it is keeping millions of addicts from getting the help they need. By continuing to adhere to the time-honored, but also time-worn, principle that abstinence is the *only* solution, abstinence-based twelve-step programs are keeping newer, more effective treatments from replacing the old and ineffective treatments that we used before we knew any better. Additionally, many people who might benefit from treatment decide not to seek help because they already "know" that treatment will entail referral to a twelve-step program whose ideas they have already rejected. Yes, twelve-step programs have probably helped millions of people. Yes, it's true they have a history of being the most effective therapy ever used, but they also have had a 70-year head start! We could similarly assert that horses are a better proven and more effective form of transportation than the airplane, as the number of people carried by horses since the beginning of time would possibly outnumber the number of people transported by airplanes in the last 100 years.

With all the medical and technological advancements we've made, it seems ridiculous that a 70-year-old faith-based treatment could survive as the preferred addiction treatment method. There is not a single other field of medicine that uses 70-year-old treatments.

Imagine if we were confined to use other medical treatments of the 1930s; we would still be cutting off infected limbs and we would be without most of the medicines that we take for granted. We don't use such primitive medical methods to treat any other disease. Why should we make an exception for addiction?

Twelve-step programs often utilize rehab as their primary method of change. Many people don't know what happens in rehab and perceive it mostly as a sort of magical process that cures everything wrong with an addict. In reality, the goal of twelve-step programs is complete and total abstinence. This made a great deal of sense in 1939, when there seemed to be no way to control the alcoholic's cravings other than by removing alcohol entirely. According to the twelve-step program, removing alcohol entails subscribing to the first three steps: admitting that one is powerless, accepting a higher power (usually God), and turning one's life over to His will.

These programs were meant to be a means to an end, not the end goal themselves. If we had another method to control the cravings caused by alcohol, like a medication, we might not need abstinence as a goal, nor a twelve-step program as a means of getting there. In 1939, the only choice for many alcoholics was the doom of an alcoholic death or the choice to live on a spiritual basis as outlined in the twelve steps. In 1939, the only option for a person with an infected wound on his leg was to die of gangrene or face amputation. Fortunately, today we have other options for both of these illnesses.

No one can imagine telling cancer or heart disease patients that they are powerless over their disease and they need to turn their lives and wills over to the care of a higher power, yet this is what most people will tell someone suffering from the disease of addiction. Even most health care professionals don't understand what is involved with a twelve-step program. They mistakenly believe that a referral to a twelve-step program is a referral for counseling, which it is not. Addiction is not a lifestyle. Addiction is not a weakness. Addiction is not a choice. Addiction is a disease. We need to treat it like one. Twelve-step programs do not.

Chapter 5: The Truth About Addiction

I felt my addiction was because of my own personal weakness and I thought it was something I should overcome. At this point, I know that it certainly is a behavioral problem, but it's also a biochemical problem. It's something I see throughout my family. Something that's genetically handed down to you. I guess I got to the point where I realized that maybe the genetic part isn't my fault but it does become my responsibility to do something about it.

◈

The perception I had about the addiction before I got treatment was that I'll take care of it. I'll find a way to overcome it. What I didn't know about the addiction that I know now is how cunning and baffling it is and how it talks to you every day and tells you everything is okay. You can do one or two, you can stop, but that's not the case. I found out real quick.

◈

I would doctor shop, hospital shop. You name it, I did it to get them. When I couldn't get them from the hospital anymore I started buying them from anybody. Anybody and everybody. Then I started running out of money. I started taking money from work, from the house, money for bills. Anything to get them. When that didn't work anymore, I started to make my own prescriptions up on the computer and that worked quite well for a long time. I finally had had enough. I had stolen, lied, cheated, and destroyed my family.

◈

My addiction was ruling every second of my life. It was hard for me to do or go anywhere without getting high first. Everywhere I went, I had to make sure I had some extra pills in case I started craving. I really missed out on a lot of things while I was using. I spent most of my time all alone in my room getting high in my own little fragile world. I spent about two years of my life struggling on and off with my addiction, I tried so many times to get clean.

Addiction really is a disease. It is a biochemical problem that can actually be measured in the brain and demonstrated by scientific methods. It is affected by genetic predisposition and like many other diseases, it can be treated effectively with medicines. Do we understand everything there is to know about the disease of addiction? Do we know the exact mechanism? Can we explain every facet of its expression? Absolutely not. But that doesn't mean that it is not a disease, it just means that we have more to learn.

Is addiction heavily influenced by environmental factors? Certainly environment and exposure have a great deal to do with the development of addiction, just as obesity influences the development of diabetes and environment and smoking influence the development of asthma. It is not true, however, that environment is completely responsible for addiction, as some medical professionals would have you believe. Addicted parents, exposure to drugs and peer pressure are all factors in addiction. There are other factors as well, and these other factors are the root of the disease which provide us clues on how to treat the disease.

Does everyone believe that addiction is a disease? Certainly not, but that doesn't change the fact that it is a disease. For countless centuries, people believed that the sun orbited around the Earth. That was certainly the way it looked and there was no obvious visible evidence to the contrary. Then, when scientific evidence surfaced that stated the Earth revolved around the sun, people were skeptical and refused to believe it because it went so radically against what they had been taught to think. Today, of course, we know better. Still, the example is a haunting one. If we are capable of believing such a massive optical illusion, what else are we capable of believing without scientific evidence to guide us? Addiction is a disease. We have tested it, proven it and confirmed it. Our society believes that it is a behavior, but that doesn't make the truth of the matter any less true.

The disease of addiction affects the brain's reward system. This part of the brain is called the mesolimbic pathway and involves several areas of the brain with long names that do not need to be discussed in detail here. The function of this pathway is to tell our brain what is valuable and necessary for us to survive. It deals with our most basic and instinctual desires, the ones that kept us alive long before we evolved enough to speak, think or invent. The mesolimbic system governs our animal instincts like fear, hunger, rage and sexual desire.

The idea of the existence of this embedded reward system is not new. Freud, the father of modern psychology, called it the id and made it responsible for all the aggression and hungers that are more animal than human. What *is* new, is our ability to define the physical parameters of this area with advanced neural imaging studies and begin to understand how this area functions on a biochemical basis.

The Neurochemistry of Addiction:

Addiction is a disease of the brain. To understand addiction we must first understand how addictive chemicals affect the brain.

The brain is composed of nerve cells called neurons (figure 1). These neurons create an intricate web through our brains that make up our neural network. The signals traveling through this network are primarily electrical in nature, much like the signals traveling through the network of a computer. However, there is a significant difference in the structure of our brains compared to that of a computer. The "wires" of our neural network do not actually touch each other.

When we look closely (figure 1 inset) at the point where two neurons in our brain come together, we find that, unlike an electrical circuit where wires need to touch each other to transmit a signal, our neurons do not have a direct communication link with each other. Rather, there is a slight gap between the cells that we call the synapse.

Figure 1. The Neurons and Synapse

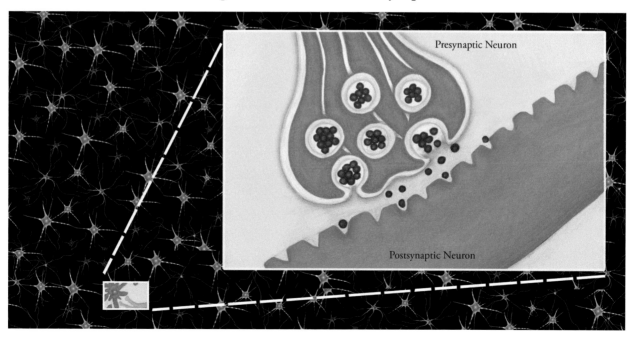

The synapse is the basic functioning unit of the brain. Which synapses and areas of our brain carry signals at one time or another determine how we think and feel. The adaptability of the synapse is responsible for the fact that we can learn and develop new behaviors, unlike a computer which is hard-wired in one specific structure and is unable to change. Our nerve cells communicate with each other across a synapse by the use of chemical messengers which we call neurotransmitters. Thus, the basis of our brain function is neurochemical, rather than simply electrical.

When one cell of our brain needs to send a signal to another cell, the sending cell, or presynaptic neuron, does so by dumping small molecules, called the neurotransmitters, into the area between the cells. The area is known as the synaptic gap (figure 2). These molecules diffuse across the synaptic gap and interact with the receiving cell, or postsynaptic neuron. This interaction at the postsynaptic neuron causes a specific type of signal to be generated, which is then sent across the postsynaptic cell until it reaches the next synapse and the process repeats itself. All of our thoughts, feelings and actions are created in this way.

Figure 2. Neurotransmitters

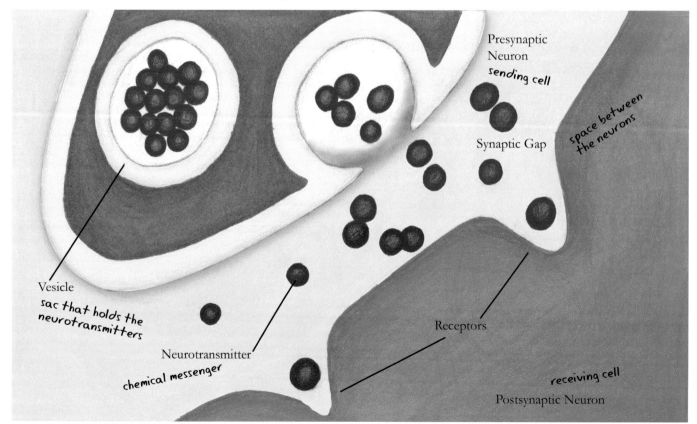

Neurotransmitters reaching the postsynaptic cell are only able to trigger a signal in that cell if they interact with specific sites designed to receive their input, much like an antenna receiving a radio signal. These sites are called receptors.

When a neurotransmitter molecule interacts with a receptor site on the postsynaptic cell, it triggers a signal by throwing a molecular switch, much like a key would open a lock. If there are no receptors on the postsynaptic cell to receive the neurotransmitters, a signal cannot be generated. Similarly, the more receptors there are to receive the neurotransmitters, the stronger and more intense the signal generated. The balance between the number of neurotransmitters and receptors in various areas of the brain is the underlying biochemical mechanism of addiction.

There is generally a balance between the number of receptor sites available and the amount of neurotransmitters typically present in a specific synapse (figure 3). If only a small amount of neurotransmitters are present, the brain will only create a few receptor sites; it avoids creating so many that some will sit idle. On the other hand, the brain will always try to have enough receptor sites to handle the typical neurotransmitter load. For the sake of discussion, let's assume that this balance in a normal, unaddicted brain is about 50 percent.

Figure 3. Normal Receptor Balance

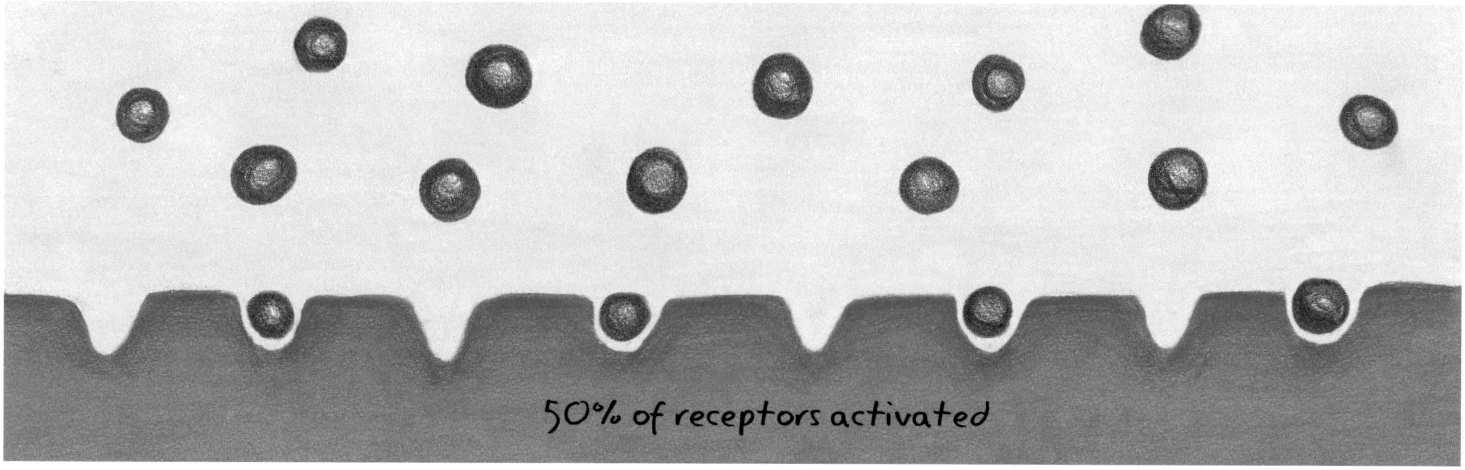

50% of receptors activated

Thus, in the normal brain, in any particular synapse, at any given time, approximately 50 percent of the receptors present might be activated by neurotransmitters. This balance assures that the postsynaptic cell has sufficient receptors to handle any increase in neurotransmitters, but at the same time it does not have large numbers of open, unused, and idle receptors.

There are billions of chemical compounds in the world. Only a tiny fraction of them have the potential to be addictive chemicals in the human brain. Addictive drugs work because they have a chemical structure very similar to that of our natural neurotransmitters and can fool receptor sites into responding to them just as they would respond to our native neurochemicals. When an individual's brain is exposed to an addictive drug, their synapses react as though flooded with neurotransmitters, sending out appropriate signals. The brain is fooled by the clever imitation, unable to tell the difference between natural neurotransmitters and mimicking drugs.

Flooding the synapses results in flooding all open available receptor sites (figure 4). The cell is stimulated with 100 percent of receptor sites activated and it sends out a strong signal to the rest of the brain. In the case of addictive drugs, this signal is one of pleasure and reward which causes intoxication, or a high.

Figure 4. Drug use/Intoxication

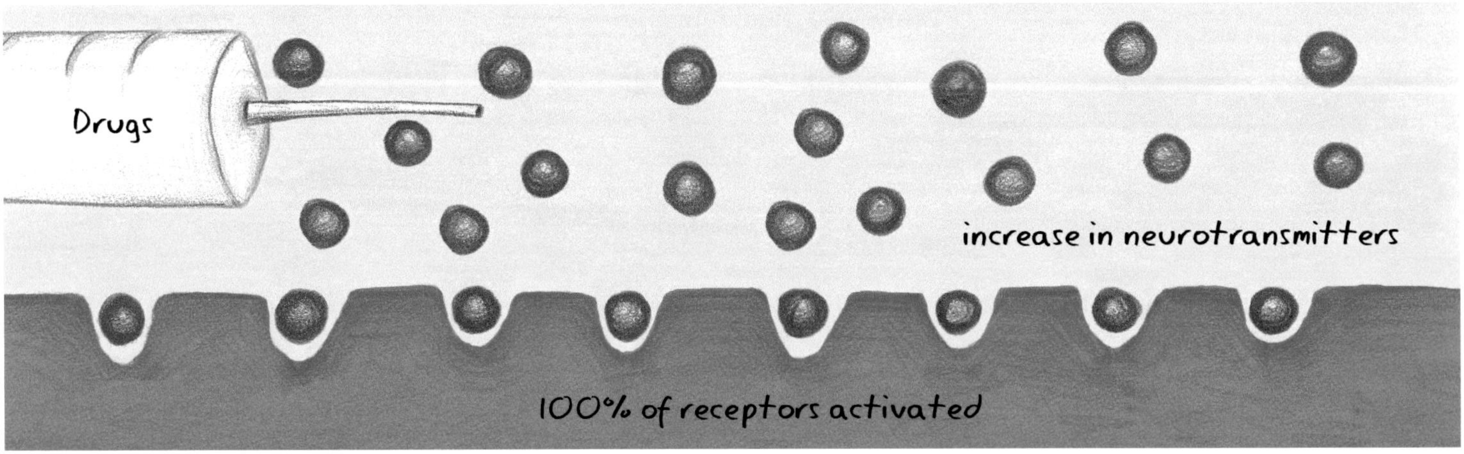

Drugs

increase in neurotransmitters

100% of receptors activated

These pleasure signals sent out by the hijacked cells overtake the normal function of the mesolimbic pathway and activate the brain's reward system. The stimulated cells react to drugs the way they would react to food or sex; they tell the rest of the brain that the behavior - in this case, taking drugs - is a desirable one that should be continued.

The exact nature of this effect is dependent on what specific neurons or areas of the brain are activated. The brain of a person addicted to narcotics, like heroin, is seeking a different effect or sensation than someone addicted to cocaine, alcohol or methamphetamine. People who suffer from the disease of addiction generally are able to "select" the exact drug or combination of drugs that produce the specific desirable effect their brains have instructed them to seek.

As previously noted, the human brain and its systems of synapses are highly adaptable. Speaking from an evolutionary standpoint, this is a good thing; it enabled our ancestors to adapt to a changing environment and survive in various difficult conditions. In this case, however, adaptability is the addicted victim's downfall. After repeated exposure to a specific drug and a repeated flooding of the synaptic receptors, the cells in question will change to accommodate the higher level of neurotransmitters. They do this by creating more receptor sites, so that the balance of chemicals to receptor sites is restored.

This restoring of the balance at the synapse that existed before the drug exposure is called upregulation (figure 5). This means that the amount of drug which originally saturated all the receptors is no longer enough, because there are more receptors to saturate. This causes what drug users know as tolerance- a need to use more and more of a specific drug to saturate all the receptor sites and obtain the same effect previously obtained with a smaller amount of drug (figure 6).

Figure 5. Upregulation

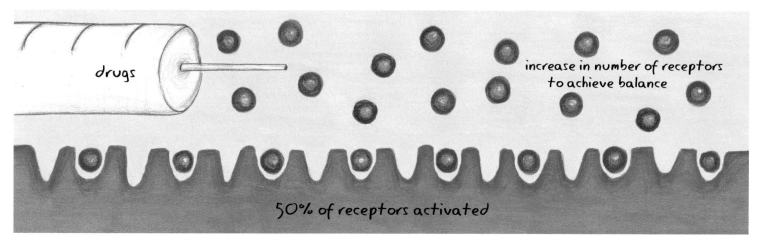

19

Figure 6. Tolerance

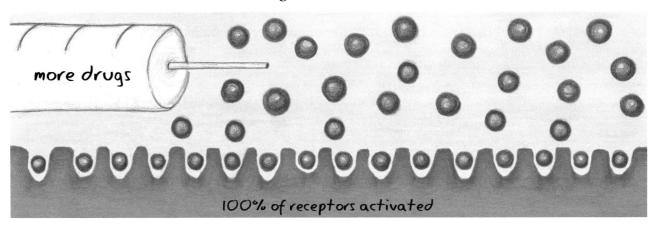

Of course, this leads to the vicious cycle of addiction. Using drugs causes the brain to make more receptors, which means that more drugs are needed to achieve the same effect. However, when the addict takes more drugs, the brain creates yet more receptors, and so on. Eventually the addict is unable to keep up with the race and the drug use stops. This sometimes happens by a conscious choice of the addicted individual, but more commonly occurs due to circumstances beyond their control: arrest, medical problems or inability to continue to pay for their ever-escalating dependence. What happens in the person's brain when he stops using is the opposite of intoxication. The addict is left with a large number of open receptor sites and a very small amount of natural neurotransmitters to activate those sites. We call this condition withdrawal (figure 7).

Figure 7. Withdrawal

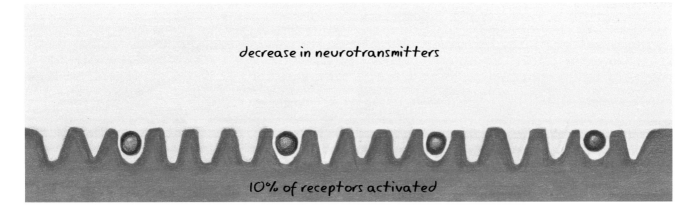

On the surface, withdrawal is the set of uncomfortable symptoms that besiege an addict who stops taking his addictive drug. It happens when all of the receptors the brain has created to deal with growing drug use are suddenly left empty. The small amount of natural neurotransmitters remaining are not nearly enough to bring the cell back to its normal balance. The pleasure system is being activated far less than normal, which causes an addict in withdrawal to feel wretched, both physically and mentally.

One of the brain's constant goals is to try to maintain a chemical balance. When drug use stops, the sudden, sharp drop in neurotransmitter levels upsets the chemical balance. The brain instills in the addict a deep, instinctive drive to get more drugs and restore the higher neurotransmitter levels the brain is now used to having. These impulses are called cravings. More than simple physical withdrawal symptoms, it is these insatiable cravings which most often cause people to relapse back to using an addictive drug.

The mesolimbic pathway is designed to enforce behaviors that help the organism survive by sending out pleasurable signals. The lack of pleasant signals is telling the addict's brain it has been deprived of something it needs to survive and the brain's only goal becomes to get that substance again. The need for drugs becomes all-consuming; the signals the brain is sending now are like the signals it would send to find food if the organism was starving.

It is comforting for us to believe that after a person ceases use of an addictive drug, their synapses and receptor sites would repair themselves by reabsorbing the excess receptors and allowing the synapse to return to its natural balance. It would be nice if that happened. If this were true, simple detoxification after the use of addictive drugs to allow people an opportunity to repair their receptor sites would be a very effective therapy. Unfortunately, we now know this is not always the case. In fact, it appears that after a certain point in the development of an addiction, the damage to the receptor sites and neurotransmitter balance may be permanent. In other words, irreversible damage to certain structures of the brain have occurred, and an individual may continue to experience chronic withdrawal symptoms and cravings for an ongoing and indefinite period of time – perhaps weeks, months, or years.

We also know that genetic predisposition influences receptor site numbers and function. Someone who has a parent, grandparent or sibling with an addiction problem might have defective receptor sites already or have a preexisting chemical imbalance. These people may actually have a genetic predisposition to addiction. Of course, if a person is never exposed to addictive substances then he will never be addicted, but to people with a genetic predisposition to addiction, a cigarette or joint is no safer than a loaded gun pressed to their head.

Now that we understand how the actual chemical process happens, it is important to consider where this process takes place. Until very recently, the actual physical structure of the brain was poorly understood. Now, though, with developments in neurochemistry and imaging techniques like Positron Emission Tomography (PET) scans, we have a much better understanding of the connections between different parts of the brain.

We already established that drugs affect the mesolimbic pathway, or the reward system of the brain. The center of this system, which we will call the pleasure center, is a very old and deep structure responsible for instinctual drives and deciding what is dangerous and threatening to us (figure 8). It also determines what is required and necessary for our continued existence. Impulses from this area of the brain have kept the rest of our brain alive long enough that it was able to evolve our more sophisticated areas, like our prefrontal cortex, where all our thinking and reasoning takes place.

Figure 8. The Mesolimbic Pathway

the brain's reward system

Prefrontal Cortex
decision making

Hippocampus
learning & memory
"Storage Facility"

Thalamus
evaluates signal
"Pleasure Center"

BEHAVIOR

INPUT

Hypothalamus
directs the signal
"Traffic Cop"

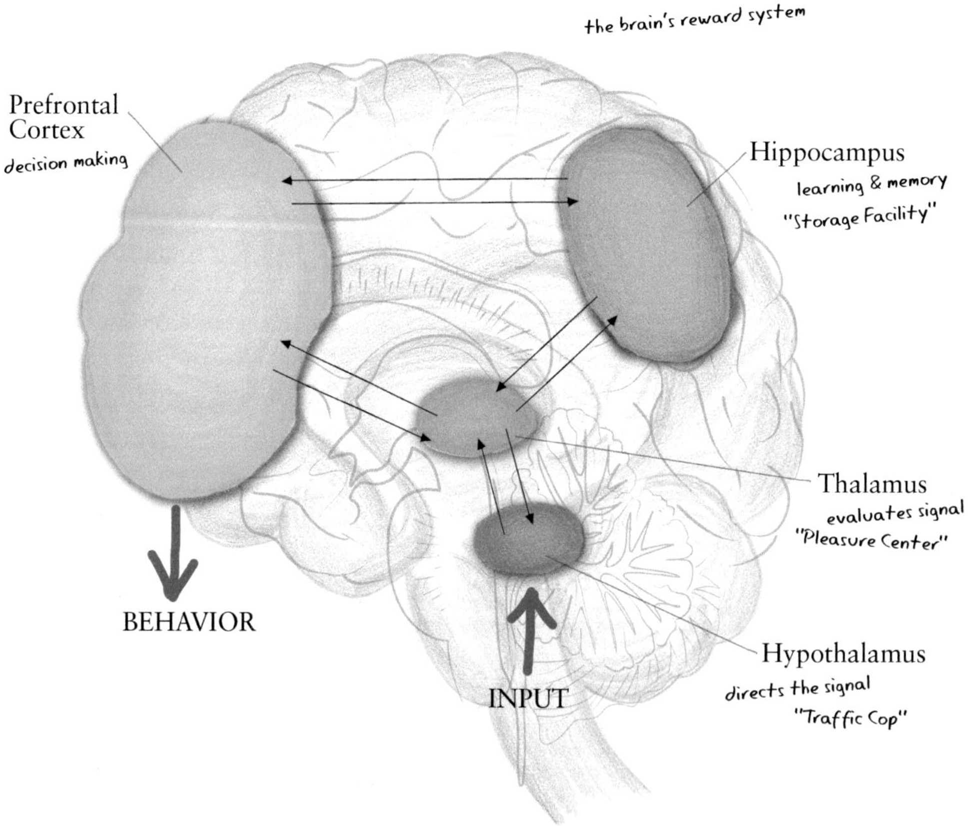

The brain's pleasure center has connections to our hypothalamus, an area which processes incoming information, as well as connections to areas of our brain responsible for learning and memory. It is also connected to our prefrontal cortex, the seat of our consciousness and controller of our behaviors.

The best way to demonstrate how our pleasure center works is to use the example of an organism, such as a rabbit, and expose it to a stimulus necessary for its survival, like food (figure 9). In this example, the pleasure center processes this information and sends signals to areas of the brain involved in learning and memory, as well as the prefrontal cortex. These signals tell the rabbit that food is a good thing and motivate it to find more food (figure 10).

Figure 9.

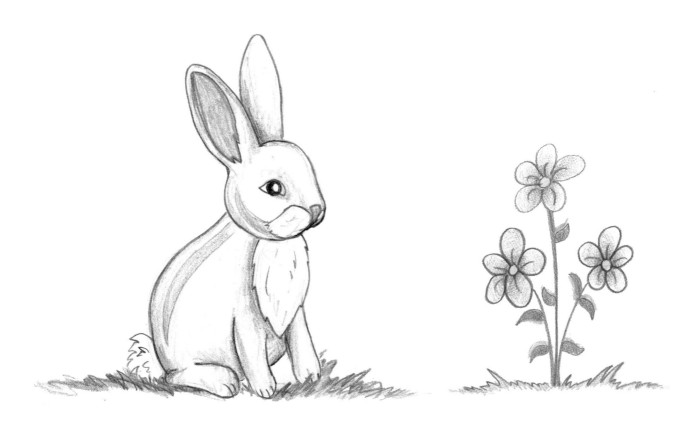

Figure 10. Positively Reinforced Behavior

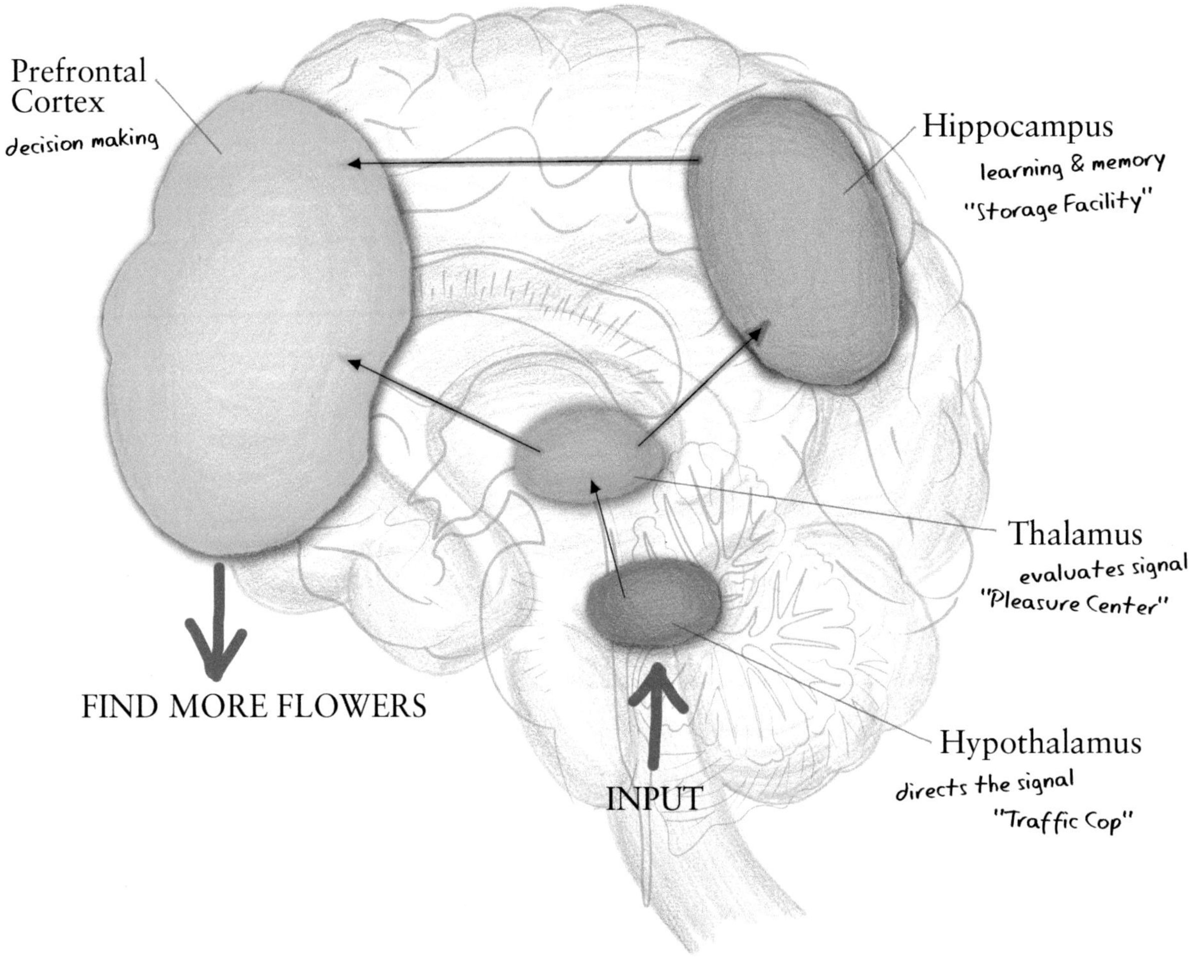

Prefrontal
Cortex
decision making

Hippocampus
learning & memory
"Storage Facility"

Thalamus
evaluates signal
"Pleasure Center"

Hypothalamus
directs the signal
"Traffic Cop"

FIND MORE FLOWERS

INPUT

In the case of a stimulus that is a threat to the rabbit's survival, like exposure to a predator (figure 11), the pleasure center sends out negative signals that tell the rabbit it is in danger. The prefrontal cortex is signaled appropriately and tells the rabbit to avoid the predator (figure 12).

Figure 11

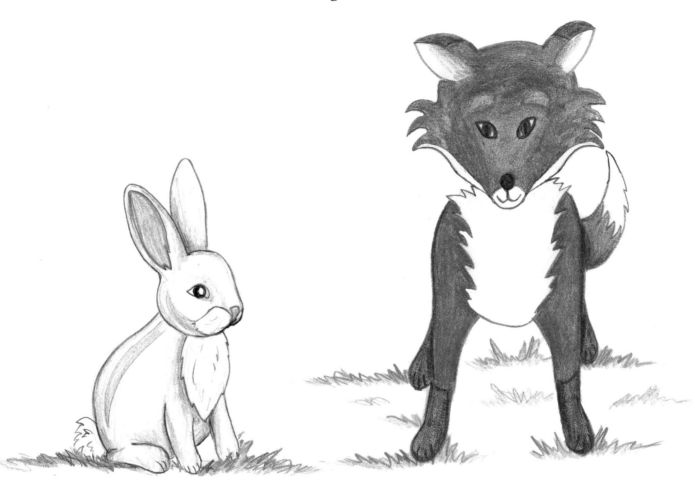

Figure 12. Negatively Reinforced Behavior

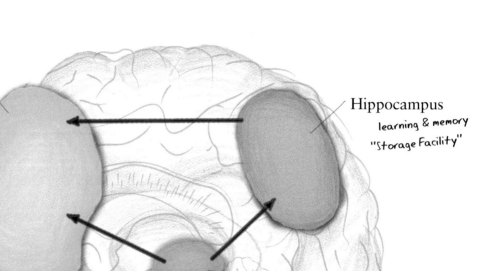

Prefrontal
Cortex
decision making

Hippocampus
learning & memory
"Storage Facility"

Thalamus
evaluates signal
"Pleasure Center"

Hypothalamus
directs the signal
"Traffic Cop"

AVOID BEING EATEN

INPUT

So what happens when this brain is exposed to an addictive drug? In determining if a drug is addictive, scientists provide the rabbit with the opportunity to push a lever to get a dose of a drug administered though an IV bottle. If the rabbit continues to push the lever, without any other visible reward being offered to it, scientists surmise that something is happening in the rabbit's brain to cause it to continue to push the lever (figure 13).

Figure 13

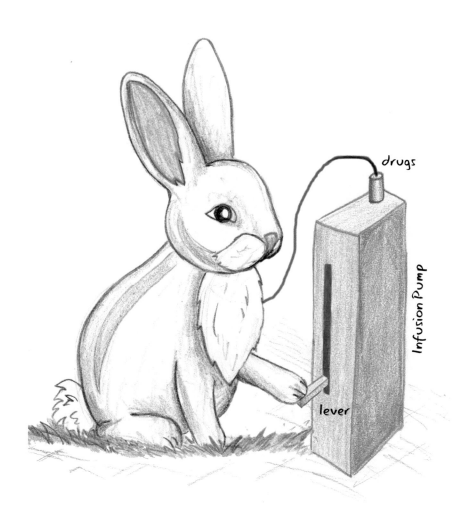

In this case, the addictive drug, which is indistinguishable from the structure of the natural neurotransmitters in the pleasure center, hijacks the brain by saturating the pleasure receptors. The pleasure center sends out positive reinforcing signals to the prefrontal cortex and learning and memory. This causes the organism, in this case the rabbit, to seek drugs for the same reason that it seeks food; its brain determined drugs are necessary for its survival (figure 14).

Figure 14. Addictive Behavior

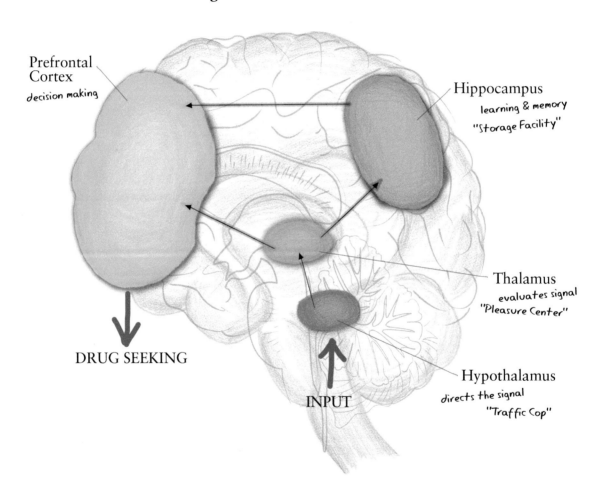

Prefrontal Cortex
decision making

Hippocampus
learning & memory
"Storage Facility"

Thalamus
evaluates signal
"Pleasure Center"

Hypothalamus
directs the signal
"Traffic Cop"

DRUG SEEKING

INPUT

If an addictive drug, like cocaine, was used in the experiment above, the rabbit would continue to push the lever until it died. It would continue to push the lever even if it was starving and it was offered food. It would continue to push the lever even it was thirsty and was offered water. It would continue to push the lever even it had to cross a painful electric grate to reach it. It would continue to push the lever even if a rabbit of the opposite sex was offered to distract it. In other words, getting the next dose of the addictive drug in the IV bottle would become the most important survival function of the rabbit's brain, to the exclusion of all other functions. In humans, this behavior can be seen easily. We all remark on how amazing it is when we hear about addicted mothers sometimes selling their children to get their next fix of drugs. Well, it really isn't so amazing considering that the mother's brain told her that nothing, including love for her child or the approval of society, is more important than those drugs.

Up until now, our treatment of addiction has been limited to supplying the prefrontal cortexes of our patients with information (figure 15). We have used drug education, counseling and twelve-step programs to tell them over and over again that drugs are bad, that they need to control their impulses, and that they are dirty, addicted and hopeless. Until now, treatment has involved basically battering the prefrontal cortex and conscious mind with medical information, horror stories and dire warnings.

Figure 15. Behavioral Therapy

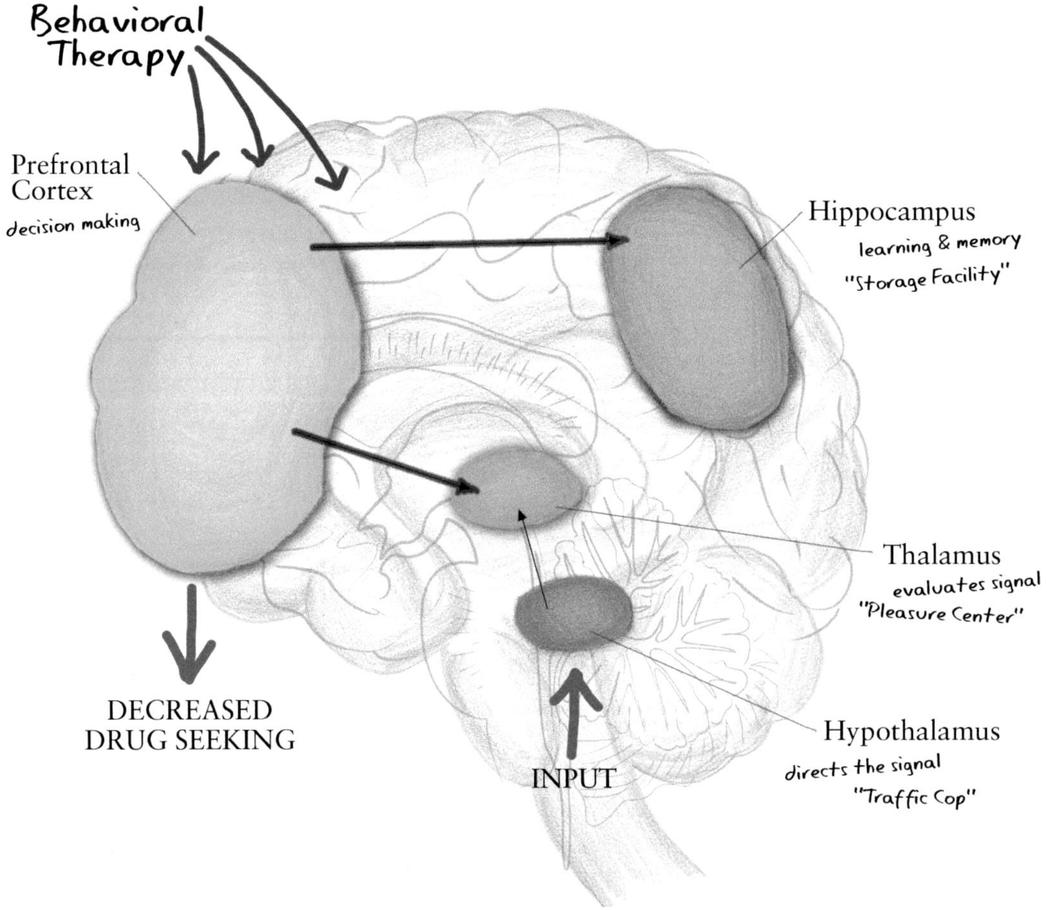

Behavioral Therapy

Prefrontal
Cortex
decision making

Hippocampus
learning & memory
"Storage Facility"

Thalamus
evaluates signal
"Pleasure Center"

DECREASED
DRUG SEEKING

INPUT

Hypothalamus
directs the signal
"Traffic Cop"

While this approach certainly had some success, it also experienced overwhelming failures and now it is easy to see why. A drug addict knows exactly what the drug is doing to his body. He knows what he is doing is wrong and dangerous. His prefrontal cortex is perfectly aware of the terrible consequences of his addiction. The only problem is that his prefrontal cortex simply does not have the power to override the instinctual drives that have been hard-wired since we were cavemen. Imagine if you had been told that eating was bad, food would destroy your body and people who got hungry were evil and spineless and deserved poverty and death. Would you, come mealtime, be able to keep yourself from wanting to eat? Of course not.

Try though it might, your prefrontal cortex is powerless to overcome the deeper, older parts of your brain that help ensure your survival (figure 16). Dr. Silkwood knew this in 1939. This is why 12-step programs rely on finding a "higher power" to help addicts control their cravings. We continue to have an overwhelming addiction problem with dismal treatment program results because we insist on treating addiction as a controllable behavior, which it is not.

Figure 16. Addictive Urges Overpowering Behavioral Therapy

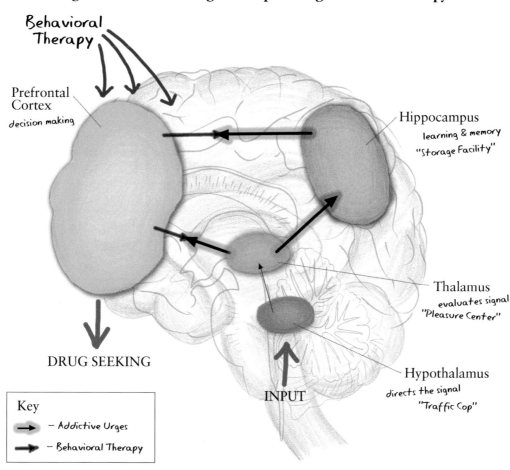

Behavioral
Therapy

Prefrontal
Cortex
decision making

Hippocampus
learning & memory
"Storage Facility"

Thalamus
evaluates signal
"Pleasure Center"

DRUG SEEKING

INPUT

Hypothalamus
directs the signal
"Traffic Cop"

Key
➤ — Addictive Urges
➤ — Behavioral Therapy

Now, finally, with our new understanding of the disease of addiction, we have been able to develop some medications that can actually get at the root of the addiction problem, at the neurochemical level, in the mesolimbic system itself. These medications offer us a true chance to treat and beat the disease of addiction like other medical problems, and to abandon some outdated ideas regarding the nature of addiction. These medicines are the higher power so many people have been looking for to heal them.

The neurochemistry of addiction is evident in the story of one patient, who we will call Bill. "My addiction started when I started drinking and escalated into doing other drugs," he explains. Once Bill's brain receptors had become used to a heightened level of activity, his brain told him that it was normal and he continued to satisfy his need with more and more drugs. "My daily life as an addict is thinking about it all the time."

When Bill lived next to a drug dealer in Baltimore County, his addiction grew because the stimulus was constant and the drugs were easily available.

> "[You ask] what I did to try to maintain and hide my addiction. I would try to find out when my urine analysis was up because I'm in a safety sensitive occupation," says Bill. "A couple of times I got caught. My relationship with family and friends and with my co-workers and boss suffered. I was kind of standoffish because I didn't want to intermingle too much and I didn't want them to get to know me."

> "I'd lie to my mother and tell her that I didn't make that much money and get rent money from her and borrow money from people until they caught on. At my lowest point, I was almost homeless, had no money and was out of a job. I kept losing jobs."

Despite the fact Bill knew he was ruining his reputation, hurting other people by lying and stealing, putting others at risk by not being aware on the job and ending up nearly homeless and without money, he continued to use. The message his brain sent to keep him using was more powerful than any external factor contributing to his well-being or anyone else's.

> "My addiction hurt me in every realm. I can't keep a job. I can't keep a relationship. I don't want to be around my family members because they've kind of been hurt and turned off by my addiction."

"All my friends are dead that I partied with, because we all partied to the limit. Usually people want to do intravenous needle use. A lot of my friends are dead as a result."

It took staring death in the face for Bill to want to get help. "I don't want that to happen to me. I just want to get myself straight. I have the opportunity to get a better job."

Once he made the decision to overcome addiction, he tried traditional methods of Alcoholics Anonymous meetings and rehab. "AA didn't help me at first," Bill explains. "It made me want to go back and use because people talking about their drunkalogs and how they used."

Then, Bill completed a 42-day program at the Veterans Hospital. "It worked for 42 days and then when I got out I ran right back out again and used," he says.

Bill turned to a medication-based treatment program as a last resort and found that buprenorphine gives him the relief from cravings and allows him to focus on his ongoing recovery. "Life is better without being induced into a drug coma all the time and lying and constantly trying to hide. I don't have to look over my shoulder now because I'm treating my addiction. The wanting to use, the urge—if I could just kill that urge a little bit, I can get through the day."

The people and circumstances of addiction change, but the science behind the addiction does not. We must consider the significance of so many people's stories and how, despite losing everything, they remained gripped by addiction until their cravings could be controlled.

Chapter 6: Treating Disease and Addiction

Within 2 hours, I started to feel normal again. Within 2 days I feel almost like a helmet has been removed from my head. I can think and see clearly. It's really been a godsend and I think I can get on with my life now and put all of the troubles of my divorce and addiction behind me. I just couldn't be happier.

❖

I'm feeling wonderful about me. I feel like I'm not going down the same road my dad went down. I've already lost about 10 pounds of weight and that's made me feel really good. I'm not suffering from any hangovers or feeling lousy the next day or nauseated, have diarrhea or anything. My body feels good. I'm working out. I'm losing weight. I mentally feel good about myself and I'm talking to people about this at the same time.

Consider how we treat disease and illness in modern times. We go to doctors' offices. We are treated with respect. We sign forms regarding our right to privacy. We get tests. We take medicines to make us better.

Now, consider how we treat addiction. People suffering from addiction are treated in 28-day treatment facilities where they are isolated from their lives and families or they may have to stand in line at the methadone clinic which is usually in an undesirable area to sign in to get their medicine.

When people suffering from most diseases don't get better, we consider that the treatment might not be appropriate and the medical community tries to develop better treatments. When people suffering from the disease of addiction don't get better, we often assume that it is their fault because they aren't really trying, haven't fully committed themselves to the twelve-step process or are just weak and bad people.

When we treat diseases, our goal is often improvement and not perfection. We treat diabetics to improve their blood sugars and thus reduce the ill effects caused by their disease. This allows them to live longer and more productive lives with fewer problems. We do not demand that our diabetics achieve perfection as the only acceptable goal of treatment.

When we treat the disease of addiction, we often demand perfection. If total abstinence is the only acceptable goal, then anything less is considered failure. This is the problem with establishing abstinence as the only acceptable goal. Someone who has decreased their drinking behavior from 25 drinks per week to 4 drinks a week has made remarkable progress with their alcoholism and deserves to be commended and encouraged. However, if abstinence is the only acceptable outcome, as it is in a twelve-step program, then this person would continue to be a failure.

Medicines to Treat Addiction
Just as with other diseases, different addictions require different treatments.

Opioid Addiction

Opioids are very powerful and useful chemical substances which have a chemical structure similar to the natural endorphins and neurotransmitters in our brains. The endorphin system gives us relief from pain, makes us feel safe and secure, removes anxiety, relaxes us and causes an overall sense of well-being. These chemicals are also involved in the signaling mechanism that activates our reward system when we do something pleasurable, like having sex or eating. Opioids and opioid-like chemicals are responsible both for the high of drugs and the "runner's high" that people get from our natural endorphins. These chemical compounds make up some of our most useful medications, including morphine and other pain relievers. However, because the endorphin system and opioid receptors are integral parts of our brain's reward system, they also make up the most significant and powerful class of addictive chemicals.

At least in the area of opioid addiction, we realized that abstinence treatment was a failure. In addition to the overwhelming cravings and loss of control that is common to all addictive drugs, opioid dependency causes a significant physical addiction with the onset of physical withdrawal symptoms when usage stops. These physical withdrawal symptoms are commonly known to include watery eyes, runny nose, nausea, stomach pain and cramps, diarrhea, muscle aches and spasms, agitation, insomnia, inability to concentrate and many others that are extremely uncomfortable and unpleasant. It has been described as feeling like "the flu times a million."

Due to the uncomfortable nature of these withdrawal symptoms, it has been accepted that people trying to get off of narcotic drugs needed a period of detoxification, during which they would be given medicine to ease their physical symptoms. It seemed reasonable to believe that fear of these uncomfortable symptoms was the main reason why people addicted to opioids continued to use them, despite wanting to quit. It was thought that after a period of "detox" treatment people would feel better and would then be able to resist temptations to relapse. It is significant to note that despite multiple attempts at a variety of programs, no protocol for medical detox has ever been proven more effective than any other at helping addicts not to relapse and return to the use of narcotic drugs. The simple reasoning behind this lack of a standardized protocol is that detox does not work as a treatment for opioid addiction and it never did.

Addiction specialists estimate that about 80 percent of addicted patients treated with detox alone relapse to using drugs again in a very short time. There is no other area of medicine that would continue to use or promote such an ineffective treatment.

Detox is ineffective because it only provides short-term relief from short-term withdrawal symptoms and doesn't treat the underlying cravings to use. With the use of detox medicines, the physical withdrawal symptoms may be gone, but the psychological cravings produced by the mesolimbic reward system, which has been damaged by the addictive drugs, persist. These cravings almost invariably drive a person to use addictive drugs again.

This information, like many of the ideas discussed in previous chapters, is not new. The failure of detoxification and abstinence treatment for opioid dependent patients was well known years ago, and in 1965 – more than 40 years ago – we saw the development of methadone maintenance treatment for opioid addiction. Until recently, methadone treatment was the most effective treatment program available for opioid dependency.

Methadone is a chemical in the same category as opioids; it affects the same areas of the brain in almost the same ways. Because of this, taking methadone will activate the same receptors activated by, say, heroin, which will keep the addict from getting sick as long as they take methadone. When methadone treatment was developed, the reward system of the brain was not understood, but the effects of methadone maintenance treatment were readily observable. At the time, it was the most effective treatment ever developed for any addiction. Opioid-dependent patients, who were formerly slaves to their addiction, were suddenly freed from overwhelming physical withdrawal symptoms and mental cravings. They could obtain methadone from a legal source, rather than needing to pursue opioids from illegal suppliers. This allowed them to restore function and meaning to their lives.

In opioid-dependent patients, methadone normalizes the defective receptors in the brain's reward system and relieves the addict's relentless cravings by allowing them to feel normal. Unfortunately, methadone does not repair the defect permanently and thus methadone is not a cure for opioid addiction, just a very effective treatment. This is often cited by critics as a downside of methadone. However, in other types of chronic diseases we also have very few cures but many good treatments. Treating a diabetic patient with oral medications or insulin does not cure his diabetes, it only treats that disease, reduces complications and improves the quality of the patient's life. The same can be said of treatments for high blood pressure and asthma. We seem to have no problem with these types of treatment. When long-term methadone maintenance therapy, as opposed to short-term detox therapy, is appropriately administered to addicts, we see decreased rates of incarceration, lower death rates, decreased drug use, reduced crime rate, fewer addicts contracting HIV and improved employment, health and social function[2].

It sounds like a no-brainer. Why don't we treat more of our opioid-addicted patients with methadone maintenance? The answer is that even the very effective treatment of methadone is made less effective by the societal pressure for total abstinence or so-called "getting clean."

If a person with high blood pressure took medication for 20 years which effectively managed his blood pressure, removing the medication would cause his blood pressure to rise the very first day after removing the medication. This immediate rise in blood pressure would occur even after 20 years of successful treatment. Few of us would ask a person do this, let alone ask him to do this and expect that his blood pressure remain low.

Yet, it is standard procedure in methadone treatment of addiction that we encourage patients who are doing well to taper and discontinue their use of methadone. It makes no sense. We know this doesn't work and we know that we have not done anything to cure the underlying biochemical defect, any more than we have cured the underlying defect in a patient's cardiovascular system by treating him with blood pressure medication. Maintenance therapy works; detox does not. It is only our irrational desire and political correctness that drives us to tell our addicted patients and their families they should be able to discontinue their treatment and be "clean" because their addiction will be cured. Of course, we often have the foresight to couple this advice with a referral to a twelve-step program, where the patient can be saved by a higher power.

Certainly methadone treatment is not without its problems, but not because of the theories underlying its use. Methadone is a very dangerous drug in and of itself. It is difficult to dose, it is easy to abuse, it makes people feel groggy and cloudy-headed and it can intoxicate them. It also tends to increase a person's addiction and has a very high potential for overdose and death. While very effective, it is dangerous to use—much like many extremely toxic chemotherapy drugs we use for cancer treatments today.

Additionally, overwhelming government regulations control the use and administration of methadone, so that treating addicts with it is burdensome and difficult. Methadone treatment for addicts is only available though government-sanctioned methadone treatment centers which are seldom in the nicest areas of town. The stigma and experience of going to one of these centers on a daily basis to obtain methadone is often enough to deter many patients from seeking such treatment and thus, methadone treatment is often perceived as a punishment reserved as a last resort for those "bad addicts" that have not done their job in maintaining abstinence after they have undergone detox and a twelve-step program.

Fortunately, in 2002, an alternative was introduced in the form of the new drug buprenorphine. While similar to methadone treatment in theory, treatment with buprenorphine is much safer. Buprenorphine does not make opioid dependent people high, cloud their senses, make them groggy or propagate their addiction. Yet, similar to methadone, it controls withdrawal symptoms and cravings and can allow these people to return to productive and full lives.

While buprenorphine activates the same receptors as methadone and other addictive drugs like heroin, it is different because it does not fit perfectly into the receptors and it does not activate them totally. Instead, when buprenorphine binds to the receptors, it activates them at only about a 30 percent level (figure 17). This is enough to keep the drug addict from getting sick, but not enough to make him high. This "ceiling effect" of buprenorphine cannot be overcome by taking more of the drug and thus, it is impossible to overdose. Buprenorphine also sticks very tightly to the receptors, blocking out other competing chemicals that might be present and making it impossible to get high on other opioid drugs. Buprenorphine removes the addict's cravings and takes away the physical sickness, but it also removes the incentive and good feelings that use of other opioid drugs would cause.

Figure 17. Buprenorphine

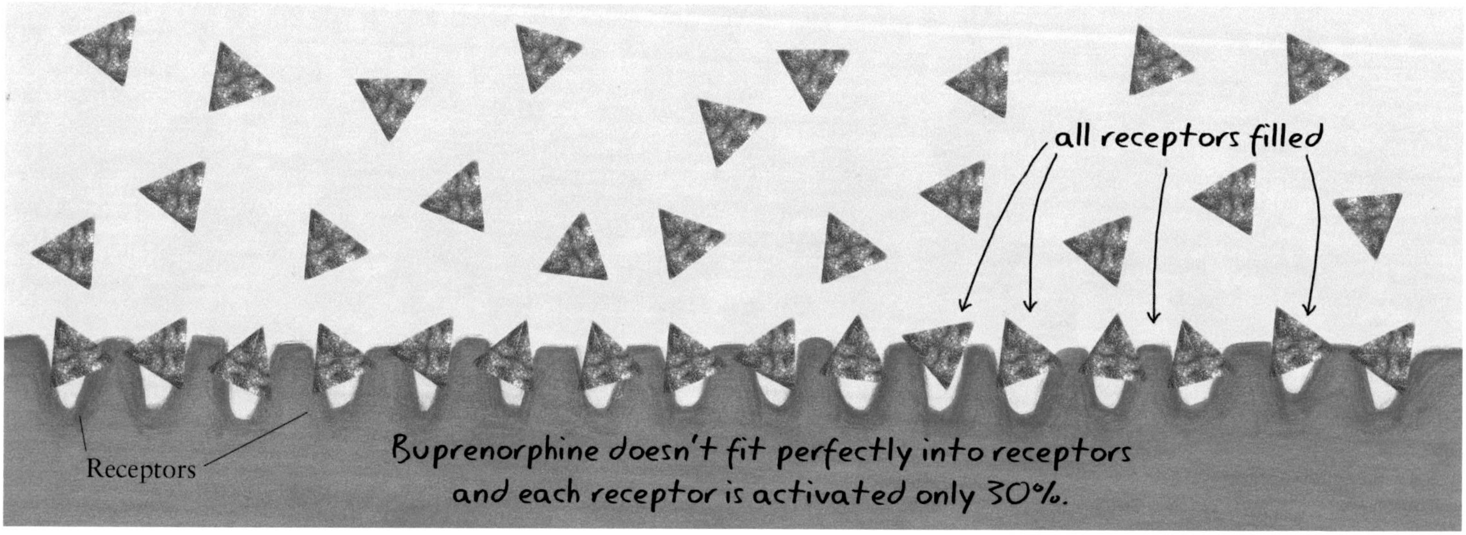

all receptors filled

Receptors

Buprenorphine doesn't fit perfectly into receptors and each receptor is activated only 30%.

Because of the safety of buprenorphine, it is prescribed from the privacy of a physician's office and does not require a person to accept the stigma of going to a methadone clinic on a daily basis to treat his disease. Buprenorphine maintenance treatment has all the advantages of methadone maintenance treatment without any of the problems associated with methadone. It truly is the key to the future of opioid addiction treatment. Along with other medications like it which are sure to follow, it will provide the greatest improvement to public health our nation has ever seen, if only we can convince patients, families, and medical care providers to abandon their misplaced faith in ineffective twelve-step abstinence programs and embrace medically proven and effective treatments for this all too common, devastating, and often fatal disease.

"Words cannot even describe how thankful I am that a treatment like this exists," says one patient on buprenorphine treatment. "This treatment saved my life. I don't know where I would be without it. I remember thinking that I was doomed after the methadone because I thought that that was the only option out there, which was definitely not working for me."

"Since I have been in this treatment, I have been clean for three and a half years! My parents and fiancé are so proud of me, as am I," he continues. "I truly think sometimes I would be dead if it wasn't for this program. I was at the end of my rope when I discovered this and I had nearly lost hope."

Lost to addiction
My addiction took about two years of my life away from me. It started out somewhat manageable but quickly became very hard to maintain mentally, physically and financially. My addiction was big enough to rule every second of every day of my life for that time period. It became a 24-hour job of worrying about how and where my next fix was going to come from – that is literally all I cared about.

To maintain my addiction, I had to constantly make up lies in order to get money from my parents, because I could not hold down a job at all with my addiction. It was impossible to work when all you do is think about getting high. All I did was constantly take advantage of my parents in order to feed my addiction. I hurt them more than I can imagine and told them nothing but lies for years. I can never tell them how sorry I am. But, I was so obsessed with drugs that I did not care.

I have had many low points throughout my addiction. One of the lowest points was when I needed to get high so bad that I stole from my own mother, I stole some of her painkillers right after she had a major surgery done. That's how bad it was, I cared more about getting high than if my own mother was in pain or not. Looking back I can't believe that I did that but I was under the control of my addiction. Another low point I hit was when I overdosed by mistake and almost lost my life. My mom came home and found me alone not breathing on my bed, the paramedics said that if she would have came home 5 minutes later I would have been dead. I remember waking up in the hospital with no clue what had happened, just that I had come close to almost losing my life over my addiction. I can't imagine what that was like for my mom to see her son near death. Almost losing my life was not even enough for me to get help, that's how bad my addiction was. As time went on my addiction became worse and I went from using pills to shooting up heroin. After a while of using needles I came to the realization that I may have contracted HIV from sharing and buying needles off the street. That for me was my lowest point and scared me enough to make me decide to get help. That is what it took for me to get clean, not stealing from my own mother, not almost dying, but the thought that I could have contracted HIV. That was my lowest point, but that was what needed to happen to scare me enough into getting clean. Some people unfortunately need to hit rock bottom more than once before they seek help and I was one of them. Fortunately God gave me a third chance and I tested negative for HIV.

The other treatment that I tried before [buprenorphine], like most people, was a methadone program. This for me was not effective at all and even made things worse for me. It was at the methadone clinic where I met a fellow addict who introduced me to heroin and needles. Most people I encountered at the clinic were still using, it was horrible, they were abusing both opiates and methadone, because unlike buprenorphine you can mix the two and still get high. I had to drive to the methadone clinic everyday just to get one dose and each time I was there I was surrounded by tons of other addicts. There was no privacy. It was easy to score drugs there and to talk people into getting high again, it was horrible. Despite all of this, even before I relapsed with heroin, the methadone was not controlling my craving at all. It just made me feel so doped and tired, I literally would get my dose in the morning and come home and sleep most of the day away. This went on for about eight months; it was almost just as bad as using. More bad came out of the methadone program than good. It cost almost $75 every single week.

The main difference is that [buprenorphine] actually works and controls my cravings. I also love the fact that I do not have to report everyday to get my medicine. And I also like that I see a doctor who I can have one on one time with as opposed to the methadone clinic where I never had one on one talks or treatments. I just stood in line like an automated factory; it was very impersonal. When I am done [with my visit] I go to a pharmacy to get the buprenorphine just like all other prescriptions and medicines so I feel more normal with this treatment than with my previous ones. It is more private, more personal, nicer surroundings and an overall better experience. And one of the biggest things is that the buprenorphine does not make me tired so I can actually be on it and work and hold down a job, it does not affect my alertness at all, which is great!

My life now is wonderful!! I just started college last year, I am getting married this summer and I have been able to hold down a job and live a normal life. I have also mended fences with my parents, which is wonderful, and we are now closer than ever. I finally have my life back and on track. It took awhile but it has finally happened. I have been clean for three and a half years and don't see any reason why I wont be that way for the rest of my life. Everything in my life is going great and mainly thanks to your buprenorphine program.

From horse trainer to convict

After about a year of using heroin, I was spending every dime I made on it. I went from being a successful horse trainer and loving mother to a miserable, very sick woman with absolutely nothing. I lost my daughter to my ex-husband, and I didn't know how to cope. I had lied to everyone that I came into contact with.

I ended up in prison, 5 months pregnant and addicted to heroin. When the prison nurse told me I was pregnant, I decided that I had a reason to live.

My addiction caused me to ruin my life. I now have 4 felony convictions for shoplifting for drugs. My family was so hurt – after the last time I got locked up they decided to stop helping me.

I had tried to quit on my own. I couldn't stay clean longer than a couple weeks. After prison, I went into an intensive year long inpatient program. I managed to stay clean for almost 2 years after that, but I was battling cravings everyday. I was miserable. I also tried methadone, NA, AA, psych, meds, counseling, religion and meditation. Nothing worked.

This treatment is a miracle. After I relapsed yet again, I heard a commercial on the radio about buprenorphine treatment. I thought - why not? After only 2 days on the medicine, I felt like myself again – like before I had even used drugs. I have had no cravings, and I am loving life again. This was the first time I received any medication for my addiction. The major difference is that it actually works!

My life is wonderful, I am once again a loving, caring mother to my son and I am fighting to get my daughter back. I am also a nursing student – I have a 4.0 and I am ranked at the top of my class. My dream has always been to be a nurse, and this treatment gave me that opportunity.

Take it from me – I have tried every treatment known to mankind. Buprenorphine is very affordable, and it works. Other treatments might get you clean, but it's not a happy clean, and for me it was a daily struggle not to use. This method takes away the cravings, and it is the most wonderful feeling not to have to worry about when the next craving is going to hit and how I'm going to get through it. It gives you your life back.

Thank you for everything – there aren't any words to describe how grateful I am to have my life back.

Alcohol, Nicotine and Other Addictions

> *This treatment is working fabulous for me. I found it really hard to believe that it would work when I came in. I felt a little nauseous the first few days but I kept with it and after the first few days I started feeling better. I really just lost desire to drink. I could go out if my friends were having a drink and have a glass of wine and not even want to finish it. I feel like my life is going to get better and better. I feel great. I'm alert. My mind's sharp.*

Unlike opioid dependence, we do not have such a great answer for alcohol dependence. While the development and success of buprenorphine in treating opioid dependence is opening the door on more research in this area, we have not found the answer yet. There are currently four FDA-approved treatments for alcohol dependence.

The oldest of these is Antabuse, which most people have heard of and which most people think of as the only drug available to treat alcohol dependence. Many alcoholics have tried Antabuse at one time or another. Antabuse does not work in the brain. Instead, it blocks the appropriate metabolism of alcohol in the body and turns it into a toxic chemical that makes a person physically ill when they drink. This drug physically punishes the person for drinking and thus theoretically makes drinking less enjoyable. This hopefully results in less drinking behavior, but it does nothing to affect the brain's craving to drink. Previous treatment experience with Antabuse has shown that it is notoriously ineffective, and is only rarely used today.

The three newer medications for alcohol dependence work on the brain's reward system to decrease the cravings and relapse triggers that cause people addicted to alcohol to continue to drink. One patient reports, "It's helped me really not to think about alcohol. Sometimes when I was working I would plan to get off work and go have a drink or something. It especially seemed like once I was finished working, the stress would hit me and then I wanted to escape it or numb out from the stress. I'm just amazed that sometimes I go the entire day and I realize before bedtime 'Gee, I haven't even thought about drinking all day.'"

While none of these is as effective as buprenorphine is in the treatment of opioid dependency, they all seem to work to some extent. Even the 2005 edition of *Helping Patients Who Drink Too Much, A Clinicians Guide*, an NIH Government publication by the National Institute of Alcohol Abuse and Alcoholism, noted "[you should] consider adding medication whenever you are treating someone with active alcohol dependence or someone who has stopped drinking in the past few months but is experiencing problems such as craving or slips."[3] More medications in this area of treatment are sure to come along and, once again, the main obstacle to helping more people with these treatments is a lack of understanding and acceptance of the role of medication to treat this significant disease.

The same can be said of nicotine dependence. There are now three approved medications in this area as well. While none have been immensely successful yet, there are new products in the pipeline and, if we continue research in this area, we *will* find the answer. Surprisingly, there is little opposition to these types of medications, or to medications which are actively being developed that might control obesity, or "food addiction."

The mechanisms behind nicotine addiction and overeating are the same as with other addictions. Brain chemistry, through the reward pathway, works to create an irresistible craving to smoke or eat, yet nobody advocates twelve-step programs to ask for healing from a higher power for these afflictions. If physicians had the diet pill that would suppress people's appetites, rather than just the pill that suppressed their desire to use opioids or alcohol, the world would be beating a path to their door. Perhaps it is because good people can suffer from smoking and overeating but only bad people suffer from addiction to alcohol or drugs.

As to other addictions like cocaine, methamphetamine, ecstasy and marijuana, we have no answers yet. With the success in other areas and a new understanding of the reward pathway of the brain and how it affects our behavior, medical science will be able to work out a treatment and perhaps even a cure, as we have with so many other diseases. There is hope for a more sympathetic public and a medical community in dealing with the ever-present desire of humans to obtain an altered state of consciousness through a variety of unhealthy means. The future is bright for treatment of the devastating disease of addiction, if only we remain open to the options presented to us.

What about Counseling?

Everyone thinks curing drug addicts simply comes through counseling. This sounds nice and ties the problem in a pretty package, but what exactly does this mean? We must remember that counseling focuses on the prefrontal cortex, the area of the brain that is home to our consciousness and controls our behavior. Certainly, many people addicted to drugs or alcohol may require help with some of their behaviors and thoughts, particularly those that developed during their addiction. Drug abuse and alcohol addiction create lots of bad thoughts, bad feelings, interpersonal problems, feelings of low self-esteem, work-related problems and so on. Some type of counseling would certainly help these types of problems and feelings. However, this counseling needs to be focused on real behavioral issues that may have arisen from the use of an addictive substance or may have been present before the addiction began and not the addiction itself. The cravings to use drugs and alcohol come from areas of the brain that are not accessible to cognitive interventions like counseling. The effects of the addiction can be addressed with counseling, but not the addiction itself.

Specific drug and alcohol counseling is particularly useless and perhaps even harmful. Continual discussions focusing on why drugs are bad and how drug use hurts the individual and the people around him are not very helpful. Each person suffering from the disease of addiction knows the extent of their bad behavior and how badly their behavior hurts people who care about them. Continuing to force them to face these issues on a regular and frequent basis only serves to further deteriorate self-esteem and inhibit their ability to recover their lives to a functional level again. People need education so they understand the disease of addiction and need medication to reduce their cravings. Once cravings are reduced, addicts are able to focus their prefrontal cortex on the counseling issues they need to learn to enable them to regain their lives and repair the damage to their relationships caused during their addiction.

During addiction treatment, the most useful forms of counseling are those that are brief, empathetic and goal-directed. People suffering from addiction need close monitoring during their therapies much in the same way that diabetics need monitoring during initiation of medical management. Frequent relapses are common and need to be understood as part of the disease and not as a marker for lack of desire to get better. Patients need to be seen frequently and continually reassured regarding their progress. As the cloud of addiction clears, they may find themselves facing new feelings and problems they had previously covered up through their use of a mind-altering substance. These issues need to be identified and dealt with honestly.

Sometimes referral for further intensive counseling or psychiatric evaluation is indicated, but in most cases, helping people to learn to deal with life as a sober individual by making responsible decisions and gaining the self-esteem to deal with the inevitable stresses of life is the only counseling goal needed. When stressed, people will inevitably tend to look for those things that gave them comfort and relieved their stress in the past. In addicted individuals, this is virtually always their addictive drug of choice. With the use of medication to suppress these desires, people will have a much greater chance of being able to utilize the skills they have learned in counseling to deal with the stresses of life appropriately. Without the help of medication, their attempts to use the skills learned in counseling will often be unsuccessful.

Recognizing and Overcoming the Conspiracy

So what is the Addiction Conspiracy?

Societal ignorance about the disease of addiction and options for its treatment are the foundation for a so-called conspiracy. We have been told for so long that abstinence and the twelve-step process are the answer that we forgot to ask any more questions. Furthermore, even daring to question the validity of abstinence and the twelve-steps is almost a mortal sin, comparable to questioning the existence of God himself. Many professionals who work in twelve-step treatment programs seem particularly opposed and hostile to learning new theories of addiction - and possibly having to admit that what they have been preaching for years might have to be changed.

The Addiction Conspiracy is also prejudice about the people who suffer from addiction. We have closed our eyes to the millions of white-collar, upstanding neighbors around us who — for the time being - are functional addicts. When addiction is discovered in this environment, it becomes a great topic of gossip, with the fervent hope that the person affected will check themselves into rehab to get "clean."

The conspiracy talks political correctness about addiction as a disease, but secretly believes it to be a bad behavior. We would never treat someone with cancer the way we treat people suffering with addiction.

The conspiracy is arrogance and greed when established addiction communities and medical professionals, who should be in a position to know better, continue their fanatical and evangelical devotion to a 70-year-old faith-based treatment program that clearly is undesirable and ineffective for most people suffering from addiction. People are dying unnecessarily from this deadly disease on a daily basis due to the promotion of this treatment as the exclusive answer.

The conspiracy refers to a society that wants addicts to suffer for their bad behavior and refuses to accept that addiction can be treated with medicine in the privacy of a doctor's office, like diabetes, depression, high blood pressure and asthma. No, not everyone will get better with this treatment, but many will. There will still be a need for abstinence-based twelve-step programs as a last resort for those that medical science cannot yet help, but most people will be helped with modern pharmacology. Look at how many people today who suffer from depression are able to lead productive lives with the help of anti-depressant medication rather than time-consuming and expensive psychoanalysis. People suffering from the disease of addiction need to be treated like patients and not addicts.

And finally, the conspiracy is denying the benefit that more addiction treatment options would provide to not only individual patients and their families, but to society as a whole. Addiction causes many of our nationwide problems, including our crime, imprisonment, increased cost of health care, accidents, domestic violence, decay of inner cities, wasted potential of our youth and poor work and educational performance. Many people die young from the disease of addiction. If any treatment is developed that could potentially help treat this disease, it would be the greatest public health benefit ever achieved. We need to adopt theses treatments and this philosophy of treatment now.

The life-changing effect is evident in the words of patients:

I'd like people who struggle with addiction to know that it's really not that hard to quit if you take the medication and you get some help. It would change your whole life. You would feel so wonderful. This treatment is probably the best thing I ever did.

It doesn't mean that you're less of a person or a weak person just because you reach out for help.

There is still a light at the end of the tunnel. No matter how hard it seems, you can beat addiction. It is a disease that we don't ask for, but must deal with. You cannot live as an addict forever... Buprenorphine is a life saver to me and it is sad that not many people know about it as an option. They, like, I, used to think that for opiate addiction methadone is the only choice. I think that buprenorphine can save many more lives just like it has mine.

We just need to get the word out.

Appendix A

The 12 Suggested Steps of Alcoholics Anonymous

1. We admitted we were powerless over alcohol – that our lives had become unmanageable.

2. Came to believe that a Power greater than ourselves could restore us to sanity.

3. Made a decision to turn our will and our lives over to the care of God as we understood him.

4. Made a searching and fearless moral inventory of ourselves.

5. Admitted to God, to ourselves, and to another human being the exact nature of our wrongs.

6. Were entirely ready to have God remove all these defects of character.

7. Humbly ask Him to remove our shortcomings.

8. Made a list of all persons we had harmed, and became willing to make amends to them all.

9. Make direct amends to such people wherever possible, except when to do so would injure them or others.

10. Continued to take personal inventory and when we were wrong promptly admitted it.

11. Sought through prayer and meditation to improve our conscious contact with God, as we understood Him, praying only for knowledge of His will for us and the power to carry that out.

12. Having had a spiritual awakening as the result of these steps, we tried to carry this message to alcoholics, and to practice these principles in all of our affairs.

    – *Excerpted from* The Big Book, *Fourth Edition, Alcoholics Anonymous World Services.*

Works Cited

[1] Alcoholics Anonymous World Services. <u>The Big Book, Fourth Edition.</u> 1939. Alcoholics Anonymous World Services, Inc., 2001.

[2] Grondblah, '90; Ball & Ross, '91; Bourne, '88; Novick

[3] United States. Dept. of Health and Human Services. <u>Helping Patients Who Drink Too Much: A Clinician's Guide.</u> Washington: GPO, 2007.

About the Author

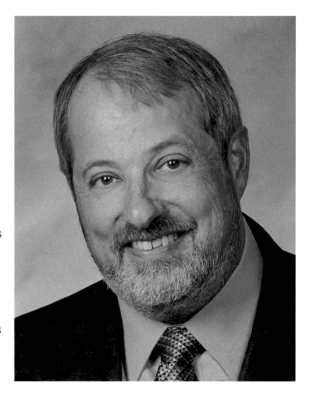

Lee Tannenbaum, MD, graduated with a degree in chemical and biomedical engineering from Carnegie Mellon University in 1981 and graduated cum laude from the University of Pittsburgh School of Medicine in 1988. Dr. Tannenbaum served as chief resident at Forbes Family Practice and is board-certified by the American Board of Family Practice. Dr. Tannenbaum also works as an addiction specialist certified by the American Society of Addiction Medicine. As one of a small number of physicians nationwide with this certification, he is uniquely qualified to treat all forms of addictive disorders using state-of-the-art discoveries and medications.

Dr. Tannenbaum founded the Bel Air Center for Addictions in Bel Air, Maryland in 2005 to treat individuals with addictions ranging from alcohol and prescription pain medication to heroin use, in a professional atmosphere and through methods that are minimally intrusive.

As an addictions treatment advocate, Dr. Tannenbaum regards addiction as a disease and seeks to treat it as such. In addition to regularly speaking to community groups and fielding calls on local radio shows, Dr. Tannenbaum recently teamed up with AddictionAction.org and HBO's ADDICTION project to host a Voices for Recovery forum.

He maintains active memberships in the American Society of Addiction Medicine, the Harford County Medical Society and MedChi, the Maryland State Medical Society. Dr. Tannenbaum also serves as an advocacy expert for the Harford County Drug Task Force, Together Recovery Works and Addiction Resources Connection.

Dr. Tannenbaum currently treats patients suffering from addiction at the Bel Air Center for Addictions in Maryland and is a medical and addictions consultant at the Phoenix Recovery Center in Edgewood, Maryland.

Printed in the United States
by Baker & Taylor Publisher Services